CEREBROLYSIN:

Evolution of Medicine

KM Schaeffer

Self

ISBN-13: 9798856356082

Cover design by: Art Painter
Library of Congress Control Number: 2018675309
Printed in the United States of America

CONTENTS

PROLOGUE

"Cerebrolysin: Evolution of Medicine" is a groundbreaking essay that explores the potential of Cerebrolysin, a unique pharmaceutical substance, in promoting neurorestoration and enhancing cognitive function.

The paper begins by providing a comprehensive overview of Cerebrolysin, a peptide-based drug derived from porcine brain tissue. It elucidates the intricate composition and the unique blend of neurotrophic factors, peptides, and amino acids present in Cerebrolysin, which contribute to its multifaceted effects on brain health and function.

Drawing on extensive preclinical and clinical studies, the authors delve into the neuroprotective properties of Cerebrolysin. They examine its ability to enhance neuronal survival, stimulate neurogenesis, and support synaptic plasticity, ultimately leading to the restoration of damaged neural networks. The paper showcases compelling evidence from animal models and human trials, highlighting the therapeutic potential of Cerebrolysin in various neurological conditions such as stroke, Alzheimer's disease, traumatic brain injury, and neurodegenerative disorders.

Furthermore, the authors explore the cognitive enhancement capabilities of Cerebrolysin. They delve into its impact on attention, memory, learning, and executive functions, backed by empirical data and cognitive assessment studies. The paper discusses the underlying neurochemical and neurophysiological mechanisms through which Cerebrolysin exerts its cognitive-enhancing effects, offering insights into its potential as a nootropic agent.

In addition to its neurorestorative and cognitive-enhancing properties, the paper investigates the safety profile and tolerability of Cerebrolysin. It examines the dosage regimens, administration routes, and potential side effects, providing crucial information for clinicians and researchers considering its therapeutic use.

The author concludes with a discussion on the future directions and possibilities of Cerebrolysin research. It highlights the need for further exploration and clinical trials to uncover the full therapeutic potential of this remarkable drug, paving the way for innovative treatment strategies and improved outcomes in the field of neuroscience and cognitive medicine.

CEREBROLYSIN

In today's world, people owe much of their modern existence to a few core technologies, primarily the harnessing of fossil fuels and the distribution of energy that powers daily life. The industrialization of farming has enabled the production of more food, allowing populations to grow. With fewer people engaged in agricultural work, individuals have had the freedom to pursue higher education or start small businesses. These advancements, coupled with progress in medicine, have extended human lifespans and mitigated the impact of severe bacterial infections. Historically, even a minor splinter could lead to a lethal infection. Before the advent of germ theory and antibiotics, even the smallest wound often resulted in total amputation, which could still become infected.

Today, due to rigorous scientific processes and with support from governments and non-governmental organizations (NGOs), there have been continuous advancements in medicine, both in terms of pharmacological treatments and interventional procedures, as well as our understanding of disease theory. Society has transitioned from a state of limited knowledge and guesswork regarding the causes and treatments of illnesses to having a well-informed understanding of the body's systems. In the span of over 2,400 years, medicine has evolved from the era of Hippocrates, the Greek father of medicine in 460 BC, to key milestones such as Louis Pasteur's identification of germs as the cause of disease in

1857, and Sir Alexander Fleming's discovery of penicillin in 1928. The discovery of penicillin marked a significant turning point in medicine. Prior to this breakthrough, surviving significant medical interventions would have been nearly impossible.

Throughout history, there has been a pattern of gradual discovery, punctuated by occasional breakthroughs. These breakthroughs led to the sharing of ideas and methods within the scientific community, allowing for input from the greatest minds in the field. This exchange of information facilitated innovation and progress in the medical community, enabling others to build upon existing knowledge and work collaboratively. However, this collaborative approach faced a significant shift after World War II and the rise of the Iron Curtain in the Eastern Bloc

THE CREATION OF
TWO SYSTEMS

Shortly after the war in 1945, tensions between the Western powers, such as the US, UK, and Australia, hit a fever pitch and began to clash with the communist ideals the CCRP and the Eastern bloc countries set forth. This essentially isolated all communist countries from access to medical developments and high-tech production facilities in the West. driving the need to develop drugs and interventions that could be produced within the Soviet Union. Doing this effectively turned medical research into top secret projects vital to national security, further restricting the flow of information.

One of the first and most pressing areas of research that the Soviet Union embarked on was attempting to fight infections without the benefit of modern antibiotics. Looking for something that could be easily produced and highly efficacious, the axis powers took notes from nature and started to culture bacteriophages to help fight infections. Without getting too technical, bacteriophages are viruses that infect and replicate within bacteria till the bacteria burst open, releasing thousands of more phages to repeat the process of killing off the infection

MEDICATIONS FROM THE SOVIET UNION

As time passed, the Soviet Union's chemists and researchers created an array of highly unique and novel medications that could be produced independently of the West. A couple of examples include bacteriophage therapy for the treatment of infections, Phenibut, a novel anxiolytic and the Soviet equivalent of a mild sedative, Phtorazisin, a tricyclic antidepressant comparable to those used in the West, and Trimeperidine, an opioid analgesic that can be produced without access to well-equipped labs found in the West. The lack of access to advanced facilities drove some of the most exciting research. Researchers turned to nature, exploring the use of endogenous proteins called peptides to treat and prevent illness.

As implausible as it may sound, a substantial body of evidence demonstrates the effectiveness of peptides. One of the oldest and most researched peptides is insulin, synthesized for production in 1921. Despite this foundational peptide, Western research waned due to challenges related to the bioavailability and uptake of peptides. Faced with these challenges, Soviet researchers persisted, ultimately overcoming them and developing several peptide drugs and therapies.

Some examples of drugs discovered and manufactured in communist countries are Selank, DISP, BCP 157, and other synthetic brain-derived peptides acting as adaptogens, enhancing neuroplasticity. Selank, a synthetic peptide mimicking the natural peptide Tuftsin, is a nasal spray that has been proven to alleviate anxiety and depression (1). DSIP (Delta Sleep Inducing Peptide) is transformed into an injectable preparation that balances a person's circadian rhythm and shows promise as a detox medication for opioids (2). BCP 157, a peptide typically found in the gut, can be impregnated into bandages to accelerate wound healing (3). During this period of peptide research, one preparation stood out, even making it to Russia's list of Vital and Essential Medicines (ЖНВЛС), and gaining attention from the West: Cerebrolysin.

To grasp the importance and potential impact of Cerebrolysin's appropriate use in patients' lives, understanding peptides, their biomechanics, and being familiar with the research conducted to date is essential

WHAT IS A PEPTIDE

Peptides are composed of short chains of amino acids, which are organic compounds made up of specific chemical groups often linked by chemical bonds. They are formed in plants, animals, and fungi through two main methods: proteolysis, which breaks down larger protein molecules into useful fragments, or enzymes assemble them. The best description for peptides comes from the publication "Therapeutic Peptides: Historical Perspectives, Current Development Trends, and Future Directions," which states, "Peptides offer unique pharmaceutical compounds, molecularly poised between small molecules and proteins, yet biochemically and therapeutically distinct from both" (4).

Although almost identical to endogenous peptides, peptides used in therapy are primarily synthesized. A few preparations are made using material harvested from pigs, which is then modified to enhance their activity in the body. New synthetic strategies allow for the modulation of properties and specific targeting through amino acid or backbone modification. The "incorporation of non-natural amino acids and changes that extend half-life or improve solubility" (4) are observed. Through these modifications, peptide therapy has overcome one of its significant issues, the problem of application. Novel formulation strategies have reduced injection frequency and improved uptake, making it a viable medication.

Peptides, on their own, have weak membrane permeability, meaning they are not easily utilized by cells in the body and would have little to no effect. This, coupled with the fact that oral delivery, the preferred method of ingestion for most people, is almost entirely ineffective due to degradation and limited absorption in the gastrointestinal tract.

This is where a range of absorption enhancers, enzyme inhibitors, carrier systems, and stability enhancers have converged to make peptide therapy viable. Hopefully, one day, oral peptide delivery will be as effective as injection

IMPORTANCE OF PEPTIDE THERAPY

There are two huge advantages to peptide therapy. First, peptides are safe if used properly, and the side effects are limited to injection site irritation. Secondly, peptides are very close to natural ones our body already creates, making the risk of an allergic reaction minimal.

Even better, there are a whole host of peptides that target different areas in almost every specific biological system. According to the Handbook of Biologically Active Peptides, some groups of peptides include "plant peptides, bacterial/antibiotic peptides, fungal peptides, invertebrate peptides, amphibian/skin peptides, venom peptides, cancer/anticancer peptides, vaccine peptides, immune/inflammatory peptides, brain peptides, endocrine peptides, gastrointestinal peptides, cardiovascular peptides, renal peptides, respiratory peptides, opiate peptides, neurotrophic peptides, and brain peptides." (5) With the range of applications that have already been proven and the great results that it has brought about are surely just the beginning

CEREBROLYSIN: ALL YOU NEED TO KNOW

What is it?

Cerebrolysin is made up of a mixture of enzymatically treated peptides derived from pigs, including brain-derived neurotrophic factor (BDNF), glial cell line-derived neurotrophic factor (GDNF), nerve growth factor (NGF), and ciliary neurotrophic factor (CNTF). It is packaged in glass ampoules of 2, 5, or 10 ml. The peptides are suspended in a solution consisting of 0.9% sodium chloride, Ringer's solution (Na+ – 153.98 mmol/l, Ca2+ – 2.74 mmol/l, K+ – 4.02 mmol/l, Cl- –163.48 mmol/l), and a 5% glucose solution.

The solution is typically administered intramuscularly (up to 5 ml), intravenously (up to 10 ml), or intravenously by slow infusion over 10 minutes (10 to 50 ml). Dosages and the duration of treatment depend entirely on the nature and severity of the disease and other comorbidities. The recommended optimal course of treatment is 10-20 days of daily injections.

Important Note: Dosages of 10 to 50 ml are possible but are recommended only through slow intravenous infusions after standard infusion solutions (do not mix with anything other than saline). The infusion should last close to 60 minutes—there is no need to rush. If the process is hurried, one can expect a strong feeling of heat, sweating, or dizziness; in some cases, heart palpitations or arrhythmias can occur.

Guidelines for Usage:

These guidelines are provided in the Cerebrolysin medical pamphlet regarding dosages for various illnesses.

Acute states (ischemic stroke, traumatic brain injury, complications after neurosurgical operations): 10 to 50 ml.

Residual period (cerebral stroke and traumatic damage of the brain and spinal cord): 5 to 50 ml.

Psycho-organic syndrome and depression: 5 to 30 ml.

Alzheimer's disease, dementia of vascular and combined Alzheimer's-vascular genesis: 5 to 30 ml (1 cycle: 5 days weekly/4 weeks (2-4 cycles per year)).

In neuropediatric practice: 0.1-0.2 ml / kg.

Treatment courses can be repeated to enhance effectiveness. As long as the patient benefits from the first round and wishes to continue, periodic dosage administrations can be reduced to 2 times a week.

CEREBROLYSIN: A CLOSER LOOK AT ITS COMPONENTS

Cerebrolysin is a medication composed of four enzymatically treated peptides derived from a natural source, extracted from pig brains, and suspended in a sterile solution for infusion. The four peptides that constitute this drug are brain-derived neurotrophic factor (BDNF), glial cell line-derived neurotrophic factor (GDNF), nerve growth factor (NGF), and ciliary neurotrophic factor (CNTF).

In any discussion about Cerebrolysin, it is crucial to note that understanding how to treat the peptides to create the medication is as important as the actual constituents. Discovering the pathways that enable enzymatical treatment is key to the effectiveness of the entire medication. Peptides can be delicate and are often destroyed before the body can uptake untreated peptides and transport them to where they are needed, such as getting into the blood and moving to the central and peripheral nervous system. Without treating the peptides, Cerebrolysin would have little effect in the infusion area and no systemic impact.

The first of these treated peptides is brain-derived neurotrophic factor (BDNF), a key molecule involved in neuroplasticity, especially in areas of the brain related to learning and memory. BDNF has been shown to play a crucial role in the storage of memories by increasing the number, size, and complexity of dendritic spines (6) and enhancing neurogenesis through changes in cell survival (7) and creation (8).

The second treated peptide is glial cell line-derived neurotrophic factor (GDNF), a small protein that strongly promotes the survival of various types of neurons. It plays an essential role in promoting the survival and differentiation of dopaminergic neurons and prevents apoptosis (programmed self-destruction) of motor neurons induced by axotomy, the cutting, or severing of an axon (11).

The third component is nerve growth factor (NGF) (9), a neurotrophic factor and neuropeptide primarily involved in regulating target neuron growth, maintenance, proliferation, and survival (10).

Lastly, we have ciliary neurotrophic factor (CNTF), a hypothalamic neuropeptide that acts as a potent survival factor for neurons and oligodendrocytes and may be relevant in reducing tissue destruction during inflammatory attacks (9).

Effects of Cerebrolysin

- Inhibiting or minimizing cell death rate (apoptosis), potentially improving various brain disorders.

- Enhancing synaptic plasticity.

- Inducing neurogenesis, the development of new nerve cells, especially necessary for the hippocampus to enhance the memory formation process.

- Augmenting the proliferation, differentiation, and migration of stem cells contributing to neurogenesis.

- Inducing stem cell proliferation in the brain.

- Promoting synaptic repair in the hippocampus region, leading to overall enhancement of neurotransmission.

Cerebrolysin: Historical usage

For the vast majority of the time this medication has been available, its primary target audience has remained relatively the same: geriatrics. And it is easy to see why, as the first common uses of Cerebrolysin were in treating diseases like cerebral atherosclerosis (12), traumatic brain injuries, and dementia (13). All of these applications have demonstrated a positive track record since the 1970s and led to Cerebrolysin being added to the Russian list of Vital and Essential Medicines.

Doctors began to experiment in the hopes of finding other applications. Noticing Cerebrolysin's effectiveness in treating age- and trauma-related issues, they started experimenting with various other neurological problems. Some diseases that were tested and found to have varying levels of success included "brain atrophy, cerebral palsy, kernicterus, and agenesis of the corpus callosum, idiopathic mental retardation, pediatric juvenile spinal muscular atrophy, Charcot Marie Tooth disease, autism caused by open spina bifida, and Rett syndrome" (14).

Despite some misguided attempts, such as trying to cure "idiopathic mental retardation" and autism with the drug, many beneficial uses and important scientific findings came to light in the 1980s and 1990s

THE NEW FACE FOR
AN OLD MEDICATION

In recent years, there has been a considerable surge in the number of people looking for alternatives or adjuncts to our current Western standard of care. With this, peptide therapies of all kinds have gained traction as treatments that can be highly beneficial and effective while retaining a great deal of safety due to the low occurrence of side effects with many treatments. Based on past experiments and studies, researchers turned to medications that had proven to be especially effective, hoping to test their effectiveness in different populations and explore their potential in treating various issues.

One medication that has received renewed interest is Cerebrolysin. The reason for this resurgence comes down to two points. First, Cerebrolysin has a long track record with very few instances of adverse reactions. Second, the ingredients of Cerebrolysin (brain-derived neurotrophic factor (BDNF), glial cell line-derived neurotrophic factor (GDNF), nerve growth factor (NGF), and ciliary neurotrophic factor (CNTF)) have each been proven on their own, in both animal and human research, to have meaningful positive impacts on the neurological system. All the research suggests that Cerebrolysin could be used to treat some of the most challenging issues faced in modern medicine, such as dementia, Alzheimer's, and helping people recover from the debilitating effects of a stroke. Unfortunately, with an aging population, this is becoming an increasingly pressing issue to solve.

Guided by the historical uses of Cerebrolysin, doctors began testing it for different applications. One such study was presented in the Journal of the American Geriatrics Society in 2015, demonstrating the effectiveness of Cerebrolysin. A Double-Blind, Placebo-Controlled, Multicenter Study of Cerebrolysin for Alzheimer's Disease (15) was conducted. During the study, thirty-four patients received Cerebrolysin "(30 mL Cerebrolysin in 100 mL physiologic saline IV) once a day from Monday to Friday for four weeks" (15), while the remaining nineteen received a placebo to act as the control group. At the end of the four weeks of treatment, "Cerebrolysin-treated patients demonstrated significant improvements... when compared with placebo-treated patients" (15). With the rate of Alzheimer's in people over 70 at 9.7%, this leaves a minimum of 2.4 million people suffering from this disease with little else medicine can offer them to slow or treat the illness. It would be incredibly unwise for any nation to ignore these results, especially if they have a rapidly aging population like here in the United States.

Another area that needs more study is the use of Cerebrolysin to help in the treatment of neuropathic pain, as this is a common complaint among many patients. Everyone, from those with diabetes to those suffering from sciatica and those living with fibromyalgia, could benefit from this treatment. In 2019, a group of researchers used a chemical called Cisplatin to induce neuropathic pain in mice. They found that in the mice that were given Cerebrolysin, there was no increased level of neuropathic pain, and it was as effective as morphine and more effective than the placebo. Now, of course, this study was done in mice, and people are not mice. However, these findings should encourage researchers to pursue further funding to continue this line of inquiry

16

WHY CEREBROLYSIN WILL LIKELY NEVER BE APPROVED BY THE FDA

Looking at both the proven (4,5,6,7,11,12,13, along with many more) and possible (4,5,8,9,10, and many more) uses of Cerebrolysin, why is it not prescribed by doctors? The reason for this is twofold. First, the majority, if not all Western doctors, have had zero exposure to Cerebrolysin therapy. As stated earlier and evident from previous research, Cerebrolysin was used and studied almost exclusively in communist countries. Second, even if doctors are aware of the benefits, Cerebrolysin has not been approved by the FDA and, therefore, cannot be prescribed. Currently, doctors can't even directly recommend to their patients to consider any peptide therapy, let alone Cerebrolysin. This is one of the significant downsides of peptide therapy. It would be hard for a pharmaceutical company to make money off peptide therapy because you cannot receive a patent on a natural product. Unless the peptide was entirely synthesized, which, at this time, is cost-prohibitive, it is unlikely that a company would want to produce this medication. Without a patent, any pharmaceutical company could produce it once your company spends all the money getting it approved by the FDA. Hence, the financial motivation is not there to get a company to make the initial investment.

The only other way a medication like Cerebrolysin could be approved is if the benefit to patients is so great that a company sees there will be an instant captive market. Luckily, we are starting to see the beginning of this. Studies examining Cerebrolysin's effectiveness in neurodegenerative diseases are becoming increasingly prevalent. Combine this with Cerebrolysin's proven track record; it is only a matter of time before the body of information becomes so great that pharmaceutical companies cave and put up the money to have it approved.

1.	Zozulia AA, Neznamov GG, Siuniakov TS, et al. (2008) Efficacy and possible mechanisms of action of a new peptide anxiolytic selank in the therapy of generalized anxiety disorders and neurasthenia.

2.	Markus V. Graf, Abba J. Kastin, (1984) Delta-sleep-inducing peptide (DSIP): A review, Neuroscience & Biobehavioral Reviews. Volume 8, Issue 1

3.	S Seiwerth, P Sikiric, Z Grabarevic, I Zoricic, M Hanzevacki, D Ljubanovic, V Coric, P Konjevoda, M Petek, R Rucman, B Turkovic, D Perovic, D Mikus, S Jandrijevic, M Medvidovic, T Tadic, B Romac, J Kos, J Peric, Z Kolega, (1997) BPC 157's effect on healing, Journal of Physiology-Paris, Volume 91, Issues 3–5

4.	Jolene L. Lau, Michael K. Dunn, (2018) Therapeutic peptides: Historical perspectives, current development trends, and future directions, Bioorganic & Medicinal Chemistry. Volume 26, Issue 10

5.	Abba J. Kastin, ed. (2013). Handbook of Biologically Active Peptides (2nd ed.)

6.   Alonso, M., Medina, J. H., and Pozzo-Miller, L. (2004). ERK1/2 activation is necessary for BDNF to increase dendritic spine density in hippocampal CA1 pyramidal neurons.

7.   Lee, S. H., Kim, Y. J., Lee, K. M., Ryu, S., and Yoon, B. W. (2007). Ischemic preconditioning enhances neurogenesis in the subventricular zone. Neuroscience 146

8.   Katoh-Semba, R., Asano, T., Ueda, H., Morishita, R., Takeuchi, I. K., Inaguma, Y., et al. (2002). Riluzole enhances the expression of brain-derived neurotrophic factors with the consequent proliferation of granule precursor cells in the rat hippocampus

9.   Entrez Gene: CNTF ciliary neurotrophic factor.

10.   Freeman RS, Burch RL, Crowder RJ, Lomb DJ, Schoell MC, Straub JA, Xie L (2004). "NGF deprivation-induced gene expression: after ten years, where do we stand?". NGF and Related Molecules in Health and Disease. Progress in Brain Research. Vol. 146

11.   Sanes DH, Thomas AR, Harris WA (2011). "Naturally-occurring neuron death." Development of the Nervous System, Third Edition. Boston: Academic Press

12. Zhovnir IK, Brozhik NS, Krotiuk LN.(1973) Use of cerebrolysin in patients with cerebral arteriosclerosis. [Article in Russian]

13.   Rainer M, Brunnbauer M, Dunky A, Ender F, Goldsteiner H, Holl O, Kotlan P, Paulitsch G, Reiner C, Stössl J, Zachhuber C, Mössler H. (1997) Therapeutic results with cerebrolysin in the treatment of dementia. Wien Med Wochenschr;147(18):426-31.PMID:9408984[Article in German]

14.   Al Mosawi, Aamir. (2020). Clinical uses of Cerebrolysin in Pediatric Neuropsychiatry. Science World Journal of Pharmaceutical Sciences.

15.   Bae, C.-Y., Cho, C.-Y., Cho, K., Oh, B.H., Choi, K.G., Lee, H.S., Jung, S.P., Kim, D.H., Lee, S., Choi, G.-D., Cho, H. and Lee,

H. (2000), A Double-Blind, Placebo-Controlled, Multicenter Study of Cerebrolysin for Alzheimer's Disease. Journal of the American Geriatrics Society

BOOKS BY THIS AUTHOR

Selank & Semax: Powerful Peptides And Noteworthy Nootropics

For decades, traditional medications have dominated the treatment of anxiety, ADHD, and cognitive decline. However, this dominance has often come at a cost-dependency, side effects, and long-term neurochemical imbalances. These drawbacks are real and valid concerns. But what if there was a better way?

Enter Selank and Semax—two revolutionary peptides designed to enhance brain function, reduce anxiety, and support neuroprotection. Initially developed in the USSR, these compounds have been shown to boost memory, focus, mood, and stress resilience while promoting long-term brain health. Their unique properties and benefits make them a fascinating area of study and potential game-changers in psychiatric medicine. In this book, we take a closer look at:

Selank: The Non-Sedative Anxiolytic and Cognitive Enhancer

Selank uniquely combines anxiolytic, neuroprotective, cognitive-enhancing, and immune-boosting properties. Unlike benzodiazepines, which sedate the nervous system and carry risks of dependency, Selank modulates key neurotransmitters like GABA, serotonin, and dopamine, reducing anxiety without sedation or withdrawal effects.

Beyond its anxiolytic benefits, Selank enhances neuroplasticity by increasing Brain-Derived Neurotrophic Factor (BDNF), a protein essential for learning, memory, and brain regeneration. This makes it particularly promising for neurodegenerative diseases, traumatic brain injuries (TBI), and cognitive decline. Additionally, its immunomodulatory properties support overall health by reducing inflammation and helping regulate stress-related cortisol levels.

Semax: A Powerful Neuroprotective Cognitive Enhancer

Semax enhances memory, focus, motivation, and neuroplasticity by increasing Brain-Derived Neurotrophic Factor (BDNF) and Nerve Growth Factor (NGF). It also modulates dopamine and serotonin levels, helping regulate mood and motivation while reducing cognitive fatigue. In contrast to stimulants like amphetamines, Semax boosts cognitive function without leading to dependency or overstimulation.

It offers powerful neuroprotective benefits, reducing oxidative stress and neuroinflammation. It has already been shown to be beneficial for stroke recovery, traumatic brain injury (TBI), and neurodegenerative conditions like Parkinson's and Alzheimer's disease.

Selank and Semax embody groundbreaking advancements in mental health care and cognitive enhancement. This book serves as a gateway to understanding these non-addictive, neuroprotective therapies. When effectively applied, these peptides have the potential to transform the management of anxiety, ADHD, neurodegeneration, addiction recovery, and a host of other diseases. Their unique capacity to stabilize brain chemistry, boost neuroplasticity, and enhance mental resilience distinguishes them from conventional medications, positioning them as pioneering solutions for the future of psychiatry and neuroscience.

Let this book help you make an informed decision and act as your guide as you explore these two fantastic peptide nootropics!

Drug Withdrawal: The Science Of Healing Your Body

An insightful and compassionate recovery book that offers a guiding light to individuals and families seeking healing and empowerment on their path to recovery. With a blend of personal anecdotes, expert advice, and practical tools, this book serves as a trustworthy companion for anyone facing various challenges, be it addiction, mental health struggles, trauma, or other forms of adversity.

Author KM Schaeffer, a person in long-term recovery brings a unique perspective to this book. Combining professional expertise with personal experiences, he offer a compassionate and relatable voice that resonates with readers at a profound level. The book speaks directly to the readers' hearts, acknowledging their pain while offering hope and inspiration for a brighter future.

Happy And Healthy: Tips And Tricks For A Better Life

Ia world where chaos and uncertainty seem to dominate, "Happy and Healthy" serves as a compassionate guide for navigating life's most challenging moments. This book is a roadmap to emotional healing, self-awareness, and personal growth, offering powerful tools to help you rise above the turmoil and discover peace and meaning. Through ten transformative chapters, you'll explore essential strategies to care for your mind, body, and soul, with practical insights and actionable steps that can bring immediate relief.

Chapter Highlights:

The Importance of Self-Care During Times of Turmoil: Learn how to prioritize your well-being when the world around you feels overwhelming. This chapter explores self-care rituals and practices to help you regain your balance and stay resilient in the face of adversity.

How Hope Can Give Your Life New Meaning: Discover the profound impact hope can have on your mental and emotional health. Find out how cultivating hope can guide you through difficult times and inspire a renewed sense of purpose.

How Laughter Can Heal You: Explore the science and magic behind laughter as a powerful tool for healing. This chapter reveals how humor can shift your mindset, reduce stress, and create a sense of connection with others.

Introspection 101: Dive into the art of self-reflection. By looking inward and understanding your thoughts, emotions, and behaviors, you'll learn to make mindful decisions that align with your values and create lasting personal growth.

5 Ways to Become a Better Communicator: Effective communication is key to improving relationships and reducing conflict. This chapter offers practical strategies to enhance your ability to express yourself clearly and with empathy.

5 Ways to Become a Better Listener: Listening is just as important as speaking. Learn how to truly hear others, fostering deeper connections and more meaningful relationships through the power of active listening.

Mood Can Be Contagious: Who Influences Yours?: Explore how the people around you can affect your emotional state, and learn how to be mindful of the influences in your life. This chapter offers insights into building a positive support network.

Negativity Is Contagious: How Your Relationships Can Improve Your Mood: Understand the impact of toxic relationships and how they can weigh you down emotionally. This chapter provides tips on nurturing relationships that uplift you and foster positivity.

How Music Can Heal and Calm You in Times of Chaos: Music has the ability to soothe the soul and provide comfort in times of distress. Discover how incorporating music into your daily routine can help reduce anxiety, improve mood, and create a sense of inner peace.

"Happy and Healthy" is more than just a self-help book—it's a companion for those seeking hope, healing, and growth. Whether you're navigating personal challenges, difficult relationships, or just trying to make sense of a chaotic world, this book offers the wisdom and tools you need to find peace within yourself.

Iboga And Ibogaine: An Overview

This book provides a comprehensive overview of the use of Iboga and Ibogaine in treating addiction and emotional trauma. It discusses some of the current research and the Iboga Ceremony and its components. The book is designed to leave the reader well-informed and knowledgeable about this treatment and ensure a basic understanding of the topic. The goal is to bring attention to this fantastic tool.

ABOUT THE AUTHOR

Km Schaeffer

KM Schaeffer is an author and researcher deeply passionate about the intersections of neuroscience, addiction recovery, and alternative medicine. With a focus on exploring innovative therapies, Schaeffer's work delves into the healing potential of substances like ibogaine, cerebrolysin, and other cutting-edge treatments. His writings aim to empower individuals struggling 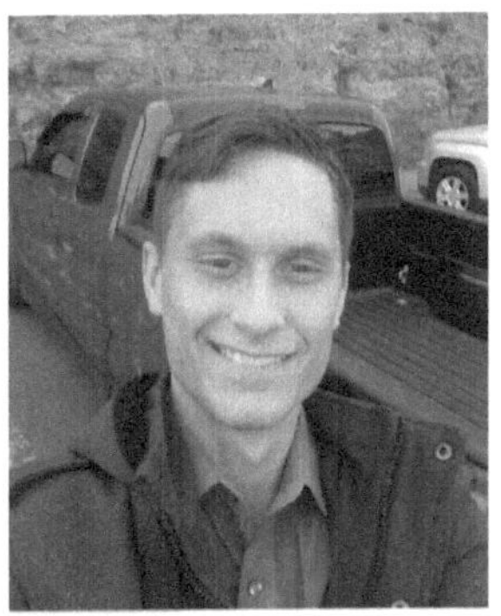 with addiction, mental health challenges, and cognitive decline by providing them with practical insights and scientifically-backed solutions. Through his books, Schaeffer offers a compassionate and well-researched approach, making complex topics accessible to readers seeking hope, healing, and personal transformation.

www.ingramcontent.com/pod-product-compliance
Lightning Source LLC
Chambersburg PA
CBHW051405250726

48656CB00006B/2285